a broken vase, envenomed

Bert S. Lechner

Paperback ISBN: 978-1-960086-05-1

eBook ISBN: 978-1-960086-06-8

Contents

To all those who read this book, and find not pages but a mirror into their own experiences.
I see you. I validate your pain. You are beautiful, worthy of joy, worthy of a life free of the fear and anguish forced upon you.

To my family, to my friends. Thank you for being here for me on this journey of recovery and self discovery.
I love you all.

Introduction

This is one of those books that is easy to write and hard to publish.

I wrote many of these poems in a single day in 2023, a day where, catalyzed by what I'd seen on my abuser's public facing social media, the years of introspection simply couldn't be contained any longer. I remember how painful and cathartic those hours were, transcribing all those dissonant emotions – grief, comfort, anger, guilt, strength – into poetry.

Looking back over my recovery, over the years where I was abused, I wish I had access to a book like this: a book of someone sharing their experiences, crystalized and succinct, into something that could be resonated with. I can only think of how much it would have helped in the healing process, to see that I was not alone, to be able to match what I experienced with another person, and find validation in my struggles. And, I can only think of how much it would have helped me see how abnormal my relationship was, that I was being abused – maybe I could have escaped sooner.

So as much as this book was for me, a means to heal, a means to make my voice heard, a means to remind my abuser that I am still here despite everything they did, this book is also for you: for you who are in a relationship that feels wrong but you're not sure how; for you who have escaped, and are struggling with those same tugging feelings that seem to go in all directions except up. This book is for all of us who need validation and affirmation, who need someone to tell them, "I understand what you went through, and you're feelings are justified."

I want to make this book as much your space as mine. A lot of these poems are quite short, one or two lines. There's a lot of open space on the pages, and I've made sure to leave some blank pages at the end entirely for you. Please use those spaces if you want to add your own art, your own words. A book like this is meant to be scribbled in, marked up, highlighted, ripped up and pinned somewhere you need to see it: whatever helps you heal too.

-Bert S. Lechner

Content Advisory

Depression, substance abuse, emotional and psychological abuse, and suicide are all mentioned throughout these poems.

All of these are serious, and can be life endangering, and support is available for anyone in need:

Suicide and Crisis Lifeline: 988
National Domestic Violence Hotline (US): 800-799-7233
SAMHSA National Helpline (US): 800-662-4357

it hurt

I didn't want to do it
   it hurt
   I said it hurt
   but you asked for it anyway
   and made it last
   as long as possible

flowers

you took my flowers
   put notes in my pocket
   said you wanted me
   until I found myself

something wrong with me

you told me
    there was something wrong
    with me
    you cried at my
    wrongness
    I didn't want you to cry
    so I agreed

wings

you clipped my wings
    and cried that I wouldn't fly

safe

you made me feel safe
    and you took that away
    you showered me
    with love
    when I broke off pieces
    of myself
    to conform to the mold you had chosen for me

giving

I gave
    all my heart
    crossed the globe
    for small concerts
    emptied calendars
    for each small need
    left my world for yours

    "more"
    was all you'd say

fear

fear cultivated
   in my chest
   distilled
   you ensured I knew
   there was an end
   compliance
   would keep me from being
   alone
   in that regard
   you weren't a liar

silence

silent motor
   parking lot
   you called me cruel
   for defending myself

pieces

you tore me
    to pieces
    your words
    drove the knife
    to my wrists
    how can you still smile

right

no right by my hand
   was possible

spark

you saw my spark
   my drive to create
   my passions
   unless you had a say in them
   worthless
   too much risk
   "your chances of success are miniscule"
   I listened to you
   I trusted you
   I let my dreams
   crumble
   for you

we agreed

we agreed
   in sickness and in health
   I left the hospital
   foggy head
   lost
   reeling
   back to you
   with incredulity painted on your face
   I tried to end my life
   to escape you
   and all you could say
   was "how could you do this to me"

myself

I discovered myself
    a key
    the missing link
    the font of everything you hated about me
    my narrow interests
    my struggle to connect
    the way routine wrapped around my spine
    the pain of sensation
    I found the tools
    the knowhow to learn
    become better
    and that was enough
    for you to walk away

over

you told me it was over
    Christmas day
    dusk painting the grass
    gnarled wood fence
    when I tried to leave
    you held me close
    with venomous affection
    I had to pretend
    in front of your family
    that everything was ok

road

an endless road
   wide, featureless plains
   a purring engine
   all I could salvage
   from my life
   in the back of a minivan

   behind me
   friends
   family
   a person I had loved
   so much
   that I had accepted
   everything they did to me
   as what I deserved

   in those long days
   watching road signs fly by

consoling the kittens
on their first road trip
came grief
but also
safety
for the first time in years

the journey
did not stop
when I arrived home
looking back now
I see how much longer
a road there was
to find peace

gray

gray
  heavy fog
  emotionless
  broken
  a hole for me to lie in
  panacea at the bottom of a can

foundations

every step
   my hand in yours
   a sanctuary
   now crumbled
   digging underneath
   all I find
   rotted foundations

all the things you did for me

I see
    all the things you did for me
    they were for you

pit

pit of pain
   ring of swords
   trapped
   nails bleed
   every day another inch crawled
   emotions in cinders
   burning fog
   you're above
   smiling over what you've accomplished

memories

all those nights
    warm air
    somnolent rain
    the far peel of thunder
    cradled
    soft sheets
    between your arms
    I can't go back
    those quiet memories
    drowned by the pool of needles
    you set me in

I can't feel

I can't feel
   too full
   or too empty
   or too hurt
   I'm supposed to be glad
   that I'm safe
   am I safe?

always here

you're gone
    but always here
    the shadow under my tattered wings
    the reflection in every face
    of the broken vase of memory
    envenomed

alone

alone
    old friends now unfamiliar
    once family stays away
    what did you tell them
    what venom did you use on them

I hid

I hid for so long
   buried my neck
   drink and diversion
   deeper into a pit
   scars scabbing over
   burying those wounds
   still burning with your venom

why do I miss you

flowing river
   once obscured
   cleaned by time
   the foetid floor revealed
   why do I miss you

fortress

you've built a fortress
   smiling faces
   success
   words of growth
   Babylon's Garden
   image of splendor
   underneath
   an oubliette
   wherein you can forget
   the times you yelled
   a pick in my spirit
   the times you cried
   to unravel me
   to call me a monster
   for what I didn't understand of myself
   the times you scolded
   infantilized
   showed every way I was broken

awake

so often I lie awake
   grief my company
   holding my eyes open
   I wish I knew
   that you lay awake in guilt
   the same way I lie awake in anguish

what if

"what if" has become
   the heaviest question
   what if I had groveled
   instead of standing up for myself?
   would I still be alone?
   what if
   you said sorry?
   could I say
   I forgive you?
   would I let you back
   into my life?
   what if
   there is something
   better for me in the future?

I can't stop

I can't stop looking
   at what you share to the world
   out of grief
   for what I lost
   out of anger
   for the wounds you caused
   that you walked away from, smiling
   out of fear
   that you'll try to hurt me again
   out of hope
   that maybe there is change

hopeless

there is that hopeless agony
   of injustice
   that they got away with hurting me
   they kept all their friends
   all their family
   people I loved
   that they're successful and happy
   despite the suffering they forced
   upon another person

   yet
   no amount of naming
   of shaming
   of speaking up
   can undo what they did, can change them
   in the eyes of those
   they've enthralled
   I can only wonder if they find sleeplessness

if they find guilt
if they find understanding in themselves
if someday
they will look in the mirror

and see themselves for the first time
and ask
"what have I done?"

self love

In every bit of newfound love
    for myself
    there is a shard
    envenomed
    that you drove into me
    a toxic
    guilt
    that if I had found it sooner
    you might not have hurt me

I need to know

I need to know
   do you grieve too?
   I need to know
   do you know
   what you did?
   I need to know
   why?

piece by piece

I think I'm coming back together
   piece by piece
   setting all that is me
   in place
   as I discard the toxic shards
   they used to reshape me

   I don't think I'll live
   without some of that venom
   still lingering

what is more painful?

what is more painful?
   is it the loss?
   not just of you, whom I loved,
   but of that love itself
   that died in retrospect
   when I realized what you did to me
   was not normal?

or is it the notion,
   that the love I felt for you,
   the touch of you, the feel of you
   is the last true love, the last safe touch
   that I may ever feel?
   that any love
   any touch hereafter
   will be soured by your venom
   and my fear
   that they will be another you?

is there even another?
    or were you all,
    and by escaping
    your violence
    I lost too my only chance
    to be with another?

to you

I can't help but compare myself
   to you
   to the way you erased me
   to the way you smile at the camera
   show your strength
   show your success

   while I drown
   in the shards of myself
   that you broke me into
   as I try and find
   who I am

the ways you've changed

the ways you've changed
 the way you say
 you've found yourself
 the way people seem
 to lift you up
 on a pedestal

 it makes me wonder
 if I'm wrong
 if I twisted all these memories
 out of grief

 it makes me wonder
 if I really was as bad
 as you said I was
 if those traits I now
 have a diagnosis for
 were nothing but

necessary changes I was too scared to make

It makes me wonder
if I was the monster
all along
and now you're free of me
and this misery I feel
this loneliness
is my just dessert

different days

there are so many different days

there are the days
where I feel weak
backsliding on my climb
out of this pit
that you left me in
that I oh so often
dig deeper for myself

there are the days
where I feel guilt
where all I want
is to hear you speak
where all I want
is to reach out and say
I'm sorry
for all the things you did to me

to admit that I was the monster
that you were right
that I'll do anything
that all you did to me
was never worse than the pain
of being alone

there are the days
where I feel anger
where I wish I could say your name
next to everything you did
and that it would make any difference
that it would 'fix' things
that guilt and reproach
would be visible on your face

there are the days
where all I feel
is defeat
that the way forward
rests at the bottom of a bottle
or a handful of pills
or something I can strap
around my neck

but more and more often
there are the days
where I feel stronger
where I recognize
that feeling of guilt
is the same one
you encouraged me to feel
for things I had neither the control
nor the understanding for

where I recognize
that feeling of anger
is a feeling that must be felt
and confronted

where I recognize
that feeling of weakness
exists only because
I have climbed so far to get here

duality

I cry
  out of grief
  for the love
  I thought I had
  I bereave
  the loss
  of those I had to leave
  to protect myself
  I lie awake
  wishing I could go back
  and things would get better

  I cry
  out of joy
  for the love
  I found in safer places
  I rejoice
  the discovery

of the person I am
that is stronger every day
I lie awake
looking to the future
and things are getting better

hope

hope is a strange thing
   in these days of healing
   what do I hope for?
   do I hope I'll heal?
   that someday,
   they will no longer be in my head?

   do I hope I'll triumph?
   that I'll look down from the mountain
   of my trials and my successes,
   and see them
   at the peak of a hill
   far below?

   do I hope they'll grow?
   that they'll find a self
   that sees the pain they've caused,
   that seeks out forgiveness,

that together
there will be a chance to repair
Each other's broken vases?

someone told me

someone told me
    I am their accountability
    that they must live a life
    without my spirit
    without my imagination
    without my art
    without my light

    I had never believed
    I was worth enough
    to be something that could be lost

    I still don't

is there another

is there another?
    another one you'll break
    another one you'll humiliate
    berate
    criticize
    stab and crush
    to fit a mold you want them to fit?

    or was it just me?

someone showed me

someone showed me
    what love should feel like
    safe
    a warm night's embrace
    raw
    an open conduit
    our emotions dancing threads
    feeling each other
    full
    a wide bowl
    whence we blend
    our joy and sorrow
    and make something bigger
    than the two of us

    and I looked back
    at what you gave
    a facsimile

held up by terms and conditions
a hall of shattered mirrors
in their reflections broken images of me
in the shapes of the perfect doll
you wanted

I wish ... I know

"I wish" has become a painful phrase
   I wish
   I knew the language then, that I know now
   maybe I could have told you,
   what I felt
   and you would have listened
   I wish
   I had opened
   instead of closed
   maybe then we could have come together
   and learned how we hurt each other
   I wish
   we could have healed together
   and both become better people

   "I know" has become more painful yet
   I know,
   no amount of clarity

would have stopped what you did
would have gotten past your overpowering voice
your monologues of all my failings
I know
if I had opened,
you would have closed in
and taken even more from me than you already had
I know
we couldn't have healed together
because throughout our time as lovers
you made it clear
I was the only one who had something wrong with them

how much

how much of the pain
   you pushed on me
   was born of the pain
   within you?

the climb

night
   subtle green
   dew laced
   heady sweetness
   fenced off
   rusted blades
   each a memory stained with vitriol
   far beyond I know
   pools glisten
   healing tears
   soaring peaks
   forever horizons
   I just need to climb
   every stretch burns
   their face etched in every line
   far below I see my husk
   broken remains
   a broken vase envenomed

unrecognizable pincushion
the needles theirs
my wings
frayed
clipped
in every fracture
in every tear
a vein of gold
raging pain
but now hope is there too

weak
not out of weakness but expended strength
tired
every slide downward a small stretch forward

my hand reaches the blades
   fitting irony
   below their screams
   "how could you do this to me"
   below their cries of how I am broken
   below their poisonous, guiltless smile
   below their façade, their Babylon's Garden
   their oubliette whence I lie forgotten

I stretch the wings they clipped
pain
strength
wings laced with gold
reminders
scars of my survival
shining in the night
making me stronger
letting me soar

I can fly
so far I can fly
and they can't stop me

one wound

one wound
   the most envenomed
   remains
   that wish
   that I could understand
   that wish
   to know that you know
   what you did
   and that it haunts you

   I don't think this wound
   will truly heal
   but I can make peace with that

if you want me to

if you want me to
    I can tell you that it doesn't get better
    forever broken
    endless cracked vases
    nothing but darkness above the pit
    the walls full of their venomous smiles

    but it does get better
    each day you cry
    each day you feel weak
    feel angry
    feel guilty
    feel strong
    each day you *feel*
    it gets better

    and it's not your burden
    to carry alone

if you don't want it to be

you

here's to you
    you personally
    you who got this far
    you who too feel like
    a broken vase
    envenomed

    you are golden solder
    auric thread
    the pieces feel broken
    but you can fuse them together again
    with your beauty
    with your strength
    deep pits
    broken husks
    it takes power to climb
    and you have power
    I know you'll soar

we're survivors
victors
let us fly
on wings of hope
and lift up others as we soar
beyond our pain

mirror

I looked in the mirror
   and
   for the first time
   saw myself

these last pages are yours

these last pages are yours alone
   if you want them

   whatever grief
   whatever pain
   you feel
   would be better trapped
   on paper

About the author

Bert S. Lechner is an author on the autism spectrum. After years of working odd jobs, from making pizza to fixing fancy phones, he found the chance to get away and start pursuing a lifelong passion for writing. Bert lives with his cats, who take very good care of him, and when he isn't writing he can be found cooking, baking, and playing video games, quite often simultaneously.

www.ingramcontent.com/pod-product-compliance
Lightning Source LLC
Chambersburg PA
CBHW071201120626
46546CB00006B/2372